The Power of Self-Confidence:

Believe in Yourself and Achieve Everything

IKE BAZ

ISBN: 9798865261520

DEDICATION

To all those who dare to believe in themselves,

This work is dedicated to you, the seekers of self-confidence and achievements.

May this book be a guide and a source of inspiration on your journey of self-discovery and personal growth.

May you find within yourselves the courage to face challenges, the determination to pursue your dreams, and the confidence needed to achieve success in all areas of life.

Believe in yourselves, for the power of self-confidence is within each of us.

CONTENT

Acknowledgments — i

Introduction — 1

1 The Importance of Self-Confidence — 3

What Is Self-Confidence? — 4

The Benefits of Self-Confidence — 5

The Consequences of Lack of Self-Confidence — 9

2 The Journey of Self-Knowledge — 12

Discovering Who You Really Are — 13

Overcoming Insecurities — 16

Exploring Your Passions and Talents — 19

3 Developing Self-Confidence — 23

Strategies to Increase Self-Confidence — 24

Overcoming Obstacles and Challenges — 27

Learning from Experience — 30

4 Dealing with Self-Realization — 34

Setting Goals and Objectives — 35

Persevering in Pursuit of Your Dreams — 37

Celebrating Personal Achievements   40

5   Self-Confidence in Interpersonal Relationships   44

Building Healthy Relationships   45

Communicating with Confidence   48

Dealing with Conflicts Positively   50

6   Self-Confidence in Work and Career   54

Excelling in the Professional Environment   55

Leadership and Self-Confidence   58

Achieving Professional Success   60

7   Maintaining Self-Confidence Throughout Life   63

Overcoming Challenges and Changes   64

The Importance of Self-Care   66

Drawing Inspiration and Inspiring Others   68

Conclusion   72

About the Author   75

ACKNOWLEDGMENTS

I would like to express my sincere gratitude to everyone who made the creation of this book possible. To my friends and family, who supported me unconditionally at every stage of this process, I am deeply thankful. To the readers who will find inspiration in these pages, thank you for your trust. To those who believed in me when my own confidence wavered, your faith propelled me. I also thank any higher power that may have illuminated me. This book is dedicated to all those who seek self-confidence and believe in the power of becoming the best version of themselves. With deep gratitude,

IKE BAZ

INTRODUCTION

Understanding the true power of self-confidence is the key to unlocking a life of achievements and fulfillment. This book is a deep exploration of this vital attribute that shapes our lives in unimaginable ways.

Self-confidence is not a quality reserved for a select group of fortunate individuals. It is a skill that anyone can develop and enhance with dedication and practice. This book is a guide to assist you on this journey of self-discovery and personal growth.

Within these pages, you will find inspiring stories of individuals who overcame their own insecurities and doubts to achieve success in various areas of life. You will learn how self-confidence can impact your relationships, your career, and your journey to self-realization.

Our journey will begin with a deep dive into what self-confidence is and why it is so crucial. You will discover how self-confidence is intrinsically linked to how we face challenges and seize opportunities.

Next, we will delve into practical strategies to develop your self-confidence, overcome obstacles, and learn from life experiences. You will uncover how to set meaningful goals and persevere in your quest for self-realization.

Additionally, we will address the importance of self-confidence in interpersonal relationships and how it can enhance your ability to communicate, build healthy relationships, and resolve conflicts constructively.

In the professional world, self-confidence plays a vital role in your success. We will discuss how to stand out in the workplace, lead with confidence, and achieve your career goals.

Finally, we will explore how to maintain and strengthen your self-confidence throughout life by facing challenges, taking care of yourself, and inspiring both yourself and others.

Throughout this book, you will discover that self-confidence is a skill that can be cultivated and improved, regardless of where you are on your current journey. The power of believing in yourself is within everyone's reach, and this book will guide you on this exciting journey of self-discovery and personal growth.

1 THE IMPORTANCE OF SELF-CONFIDENCE

Self-confidence, often considered the foundation of all our personal achievements, is an attribute that permeates every aspect of our lives. It is that internal voice that encourages us to take the first step toward our goals, to persist in the face of challenges, and to believe in our untapped potential. In this chapter, we will explore the fundamental importance of self-confidence and its comprehensive influence on all areas of human existence.

Self-confidence is not a mere psychological accessory; it is a driving force that shapes our decisions, our interactions, and our destiny. It empowers us to overcome obstacles, embrace opportunities, and achieve our boldest dreams. Without it, we often find ourselves trapped in a cycle of self-doubt that limits our potential and hinders personal growth.

As we delve into the pages of this chapter, we will examine how self-confidence affects our relationships, our careers, and our quest for self-realization. We will discover how it forms the foundation for healthy self-esteem and how we can begin to cultivate it even when facing seemingly insurmountable challenges.

So, prepare to explore the fascinating world of self-confidence and understand why believing in yourself is the key to conquering everything you desire in life. This is the starting point for an exciting journey toward a more confident and fulfilled version of yourself.

What Is Self-Confidence?

Self-confidence is a fundamental psychological and emotional state that manifests when a person believes in their own abilities, judgments, and capabilities. It is the unwavering belief that you possess the potential and competence needed to face life's challenges and achieve your goals. Self-confidence is not just a fleeting feeling but a deeply rooted attitude that permeates how you see yourself, interact with the world, and confront adversity.

It is closely linked to self-esteem, which is the subjective evaluation we make of ourselves. Having healthy self-esteem is an essential component of self-confidence because when you value yourself, you are more likely to trust your own decisions and actions.

Self-confidence does not imply arrogance or an overly positive view of oneself. Instead, it is a realistic understanding of your abilities, both strengths and weaknesses. Having self-confidence does not mean never doubting yourself but rather believing that, even in the face of doubt, you have the capacity to confront challenges and move forward.

It is important to note that self-confidence is not a fixed personality trait. It can be developed and strengthened over time through self-awareness, learning, and experience. The journey toward solid self-confidence involves exploring your own beliefs and limitations, overcoming obstacles, and building a more positive relationship with yourself.

However, self-confidence is not a final goal but an ongoing skill of self-development. It is dynamic and can be influenced by life events and circumstances. By understanding what self-confidence is and how it operates in our lives, you will be better prepared to embark on a journey of personal growth and the pursuit of your goals.

The Benefits of Self-Confidence

The benefits of self-confidence are vast and comprehensive, permeating all areas of life. When a person possesses a healthy level of self-confidence, they experience significant changes in their mindset, behavior, and relationships. Let's explore these benefits in detail.

Firstly, self-confidence is intrinsically linked to resilience. Self-confident individuals tend to handle adversities and challenges better. They view setbacks as learning opportunities and are more likely to overcome obstacles. This not only reduces stress but also enhances the ability to deal with difficult situations, promoting a more resilient mindset.

Additionally, self-confidence is a vital component of personal development. When you believe in yourself, you are more willing to explore new areas, acquire new skills, and step out of your comfort zone. This leads to personal growth, the discovery of hidden talents, and broadening horizons, making your life richer and more meaningful.

Self-confidence also positively impacts decision-making. Confident individuals find it easier to make decisions because they trust their own judgments and intuitions. They do not become paralyzed by indecision, which enables them to progress more effectively toward their goals.

Personal relationships are another area benefitted by self-confidence. Self-confident individuals often establish healthier and more satisfying relationships. They are better communicators, set boundaries effectively, and are more likely to attract people who respect and value them.

In the professional realm, self-confidence is an invaluable asset. It enhances leadership, influence, and persuasion abilities. Confident individuals often achieve more success in their careers because they have the courage to pursue opportunities, face challenges, and excel in their respective fields.

Moreover, self-confidence is closely related to healthy self-esteem. When you value yourself and believe in your abilities, you are more likely to take care of yourself, maintain healthy lifestyle habits, and set ambitious goals. This contributes to overall emotional and physical well-being.

Self-confidence also plays a vital role in motivation. When you have confidence in yourself, you are more inclined to set challenging goals and strive to achieve them. Belief in your capacity for success drives intrinsic motivation, making it more likely for you to persist in your efforts, even when facing difficulties.

Another significant benefit is improved communication. Self-confident individuals tend to express themselves more clearly, assertively, and persuasively. They inspire confidence in others and are effective at articulating ideas and advocating for their opinions, making them effective leaders in teams and work environments.

Self-confidence also contributes to self-acceptance. When you believe in yourself, you are more likely to accept your imperfections and forgive yourself for past mistakes. This promotes self-compassion, which is essential for mental health and emotional well-being.

Another important aspect is the reduction of social anxiety. Self-confident people are less likely to be dominated by the fear of others' judgment. This allows them to express themselves more freely in social situations and create more genuine connections with others.

Self-confidence also boosts initiative and creativity. When you believe in your ability to accomplish something, you are more likely to have innovative ideas and take action to turn them into reality. This can be extremely valuable in entrepreneurship, problem-solving, and innovation.

Additionally, self-confidence strengthens your ability to withstand external pressure. You are less susceptible to negative influence and more capable of maintaining your values and goals, even when faced with criticism or opposition.

Self-confidence also has physical impacts. Self-confident

individuals tend to take better care of themselves, resulting in overall better health. This includes habits such as a healthy diet, regular exercise, and adequate sleep.

Another important dimension is the ability to excel in competitive situations. Self-confidence enhances your competitive mindset, making you strive for success in competitive fields, from sports to the workplace.

Self-confidence also plays a role in building a positive self-image. When you feel good about yourself and believe in your ability to achieve goals, it reflects in a positive image that others have of you.

Furthermore, self-confidence makes communication more effective. You are more assertive and capable of expressing your opinions and needs clearly and respectfully. This improves your relationships and prevents unnecessary conflicts.

Self-confidence also influences how you handle criticism and feedback. Confident individuals are more open to constructive criticism, learn from it, and make adjustments to their actions rather than feeling threatened or defeated by it.

Finally, self-confidence contributes to a sense of empowerment. It gives you the feeling of being in control of your own life and destiny. You become

In summary, the benefits of self-confidence are vast and deeply impact all areas of life. It strengthens resilience, promotes personal growth, improves relationships, drives professional success, contributes to emotional and physical well-being, and empowers you to face life with courage and determination. It is an attribute that not only transforms how you see yourself but also how the world sees you and how you interact with it.

The Consequences of Lack of Self-Confidence

Lack of self-confidence can have a series of profound and negative consequences that affect every aspect of a person's life. These consequences can manifest in varied ways and often limit an individual's potential to achieve their goals and live a fulfilling and satisfying life.

One of the most obvious consequences of low self-confidence is constant self-doubt. Individuals with low self-confidence tend to question their own abilities, decisions, and actions continuously. This can lead to a cycle of negativity where a lack of self-belief results in underperformance.

Additionally, lack of self-confidence can lead to procrastination. When someone doesn't believe they can successfully complete a task, they are more likely to postpone it, which, in turn, can lead to increased stress and anxiety.

Lack of self-confidence can also have a significant impact on interpersonal relationships. People with low self-confidence may struggle to establish deep and healthy connections as they often doubt their own worth and fear rejection. This can lead to social isolation and loneliness.

In the workplace, lack of self-confidence can hinder career progress. Hesitation to take on responsibilities or seek prominent opportunities can result in professional stagnation and job dissatisfaction.

Another common consequence of lack of self-confidence is perfectionism. Individuals who lack confidence in their abilities often overexert themselves to avoid making mistakes. This can lead to high levels of anxiety and stress as the relentless pursuit of perfection is often unattainable.

Lack of self-confidence can also lead to self-rejection. Those with low self-esteem often view themselves as unworthy of love, success, and happiness. This can create a cycle of self-sabotage where the person does not pursue positive opportunities because they believe they don't deserve them.

On a deeper level, lack of self-confidence can affect mental health. It can contribute to anxiety, depression, and other mental health issues as constant self-criticism and negativity undermine emotional well-being.

Another consequence is a lack of assertiveness. People with low self-confidence often struggle to express their needs and desires clearly and assertively. This can lead to dysfunctional relationships and personal dissatisfaction.

Lack of self-confidence can also negatively impact decision-making. Individuals who lack confidence in their own choices often resort to constant indecision, which can result in missed opportunities and regrets.

Furthermore, lack of self-confidence can lead to a cycle of failures. Those who don't believe in themselves often underestimate their abilities and do not allow themselves to pursue ambitious goals. This can result in a track record of achievements below their potential.

Lack of self-confidence can also impair effective communication. People who doubt their own abilities often have difficulty expressing their ideas and opinions clearly, which can harm personal and professional relationships.

Another worrying consequence is the inability to face challenges with resilience. Those who lack self-confidence may crumble in the face of adversity instead of seeing it as an opportunity for learning and growth.

Lack of self-confidence can also lead to a constant search for external validation. People who don't trust their own opinions and choices often seek constant approval and validation from others, which can be exhausting and limiting.

Ultimately, lack of self-confidence can result in a less satisfying life. Individuals who don't believe in themselves often settle for less than they deserve in terms of relationships, career, and personal fulfillment.

In summary, lack of self-confidence can have a wide range of negative consequences that affect quality of life, relationships, professional performance, and mental health. Recognizing the importance of self-confidence and working to develop it is crucial to overcoming these challenges and reaching one's full potential.

2 THE JOURNEY OF SELF-KNOWLEDGE

The journey of self-discovery is a fascinating and transformative path that takes us to the core of who we are, revealing our true motivations, passions, and limitations. This chapter will delve deeply into this process of self-discovery, highlighting the fundamental importance of getting to know ourselves more intimately and genuinely.

However, the journey of self-discovery is not just a quest for answers. It is a continuous exploration that challenges us to question our beliefs, face our fears, and embrace our authenticity. It is an invitation to a deeper connection with ourselves, to understand why we do what we do, and how we can grow from this understanding.

This chapter will be a guided exploration, providing insights and tools to assist you in your own journey of self-connoisseurship. Throughout these pages, we will examine the key steps of this process, from self-reflection to accepting our imperfections, with the aim of helping you build a solid foundation of self-confidence and personal growth.

Preparing for the journey of self-discovery is an important step towards a more meaningful and satisfying life. It is a quest that will enrich you internally and also positively influence the way you interact with the world around you. So, embark on this journey with an open mind and a willing heart, as self-awareness is the foundation of a fully lived life.

Discovering Who You Really Are

Discovering who you really are is one of the most significant and transformative journeys one can undertake. This deep and introspective quest not only connects us with our inner self but also helps us understand our motivations, values, and unique identity. It is a process that transcends the surface of our personality and delves into the deeper layers of our psyche.

However, this journey often begins with self-reflection. It takes a moment of pause, of silence, to look within and question our own beliefs, desires, and goals. Questions like "What really matters to me?" and "What are my core values?" are essential to begin unraveling the mysteries of who we are.

As we venture deeper into this quest, we discover that we are complex beings, shaped by past experiences, cultural influences, and relationships. Understanding our personal history is crucial to discovering who we are, as many of our traits and behaviors have roots in our life journey.

Acceptance plays a fundamental role in uncovering our true identity. This involves embracing all parts of ourselves, including imperfections and vulnerabilities that may have been suppressed. Self-acceptance allows us to embrace our humanity and our authenticity.

The practice of gratitude is another powerful tool in this journey. By recognizing and appreciating our strengths, accomplishments, and even our challenges, we cultivate a deep respect for ourselves. This helps build a positive self-image and strengthens self-confidence.

The pursuit of authenticity is a crucial aspect of discovering who we are. Often, we spend years adapting our identity to meet others' expectations. However, finding our authentic voice and living in line with our values is essential for a meaningful life.

Self-knowledge also helps us establish healthy boundaries. As we understand our needs and desires, we can communicate our boundaries more effectively and avoid emotional overload.

It is important to remember that the journey of self-discovery is ongoing. As life evolves and we face new challenges, our understanding of ourselves also expands. Therefore, it is an ever-evolving quest that accompanies us throughout life.

The journey of discovering who you really are is not without challenges. Often, we confront uncomfortable aspects of our personality, deal with doubts and uncertainties, and face internal resistance. However, it is these challenges that allow us to grow and evolve.

A crucial step is to listen to your intuition. Often, our intuition is a reliable compass that points us in the right direction. Learning to tune into your intuition and trust your inner wisdom can be a valuable guide on this journey.

Another aspect is authenticity in relationships. As you get to know yourself better, you are better equipped to establish deep and meaningful connections with others. Authentic relationships are built on honesty, vulnerability, and mutual respect.

Discovering who you really are also involves confronting limiting beliefs that may be holding you back. This includes identifying negative thoughts about yourself and replacing them with positive and constructive affirmations.

Meditation and mindfulness practice are powerful tools for connecting with your inner self. They allow you to calm your mind, reduce mental noise, and access a deeper understanding of yourself.

As this journey progresses, you may also find your life's purpose. This involves discovering what truly inspires you, what makes you feel alive, and how you can contribute meaningfully to the world.

Remember that the journey of self-discovery is not linear. There will be ups and downs, moments of clarity, and moments of confusion. However, each step along the way is valuable as it helps you become the best version of yourself.

In summary, discovering who you truly are is a deep and transformative journey of self-discovery. It involves self-reflection, acceptance, gratitude, authenticity, setting boundaries, listening to intuition, building authentic relationships, and confronting limiting beliefs. It is an ongoing process that empowers you to live a more authentic, meaningful life in tune with your true identity.

Overcoming Insecurities

Overcoming insecurities is a journey that many of us undertake throughout life. Insecurities can manifest in various ways and can be deeply rooted in our psychology and past experiences. However, it is a worthwhile journey as it frees us from the shackles that hinder us from reaching our true potential.

A crucial step in overcoming insecurities is self-examination. It is necessary to look deep within yourself and identify the sources of your insecurities. This may involve reflecting on past experiences, negative thought patterns, and self-criticism.

Recognizing and naming your insecurities is an important step. Sometimes, insecurities can hide in the subconscious and manifest subtly. Identifying and naming these insecurities allows you to confront them more directly.

Self-acceptance plays a fundamental role in overcoming insecurities. This involves embracing all parts of yourself, including areas you may consider imperfect. Self-acceptance doesn't mean you can't grow or improve; it means accepting yourself as you are at this moment.

Challenging limiting beliefs is another crucial step.

Often, insecurities are fueled by negative beliefs about oneself. Questioning these beliefs and replacing them with more positive and realistic thoughts is a vital step in overcoming insecurities.

Building self-esteem is essential. When you value yourself and acknowledge your own qualities and accomplishments, insecurities are less likely to dominate you. This doesn't mean being arrogant but recognizing your own worth.

The practice of self-compassion is also fundamental. Treating yourself with the same kindness and compassion as you would a friend is an effective way to neutralize self-criticism and build self-confidence.

Seeking external support can be valuable. Talking to a therapist or counselor can help you explore your insecurities in a safe environment and receive guidance on how to address them.

Gradual exposure to situations that make you feel insecure is an effective technique. Confronting your insecurities in a controlled and gradual manner can help desensitize the negative emotions associated with them.

Building personal and professional skills is also a significant step. Sometimes, insecurities are linked to a sense of incompetence. Investing in your personal development and acquiring new skills can boost your self-confidence.

Seeking role models and mentors is also valuable. Finding people who have overcome similar insecurities and achieved success can inspire you and provide practical guidance.

The practice of gratitude is a powerful way to shift your focus from insecurities to the positive aspects of your life. Regularly acknowledging and appreciating the blessings in your life can improve your emotional well-being.

Cognitive-behavioral therapy (CBT) is an effective approach to overcoming insecurities. It focuses on identifying and restructuring negative thought patterns that feed insecurities.

Building healthy relationships is important. Having friends and family who support and value you is essential for building self-esteem and overcoming insecurities.

The practice of assertiveness is also a valuable skill. Being able to express your needs and desires respectfully and effectively helps build self-confidence and address insecurities.

Building a positive social circle is crucial. Surrounding yourself with people who support and encourage you can help combat negative influences that feed your insecurities.

Authenticity in relationships is crucial. Being authentic and vulnerable in your relationships allows you to build more genuine and meaningful connections.

Continuous self-reflection is an effective way to keep track of your insecurities and continue working on them over time.

It's important to remember that overcoming insecurities is an ongoing journey. It's not an easy task, and there may be setbacks along the way. However, with determination, support, and self-acceptance, it is possible to overcome these barriers and live a more confident and fulfilled life.

Exploring Your Passions and Talents

Exploring your passions and talents is a rewarding journey that can enrich your life in deep and meaningful ways. By diving into this process of self-discovery, you come closer to understanding what makes you feel alive and fulfilled. It's an exploration that transcends the superficiality of daily life, taking you into an inner world of unique interests and abilities.

An essential part of this journey is self-reflection. It's essential to take time to contemplate what truly inspires you, what makes your heart beat faster, and what you completely lose yourself in when engaged. This may involve recalling past experiences that excited you or moments when you felt most authentic.

A willingness to try new things is crucial. Sometimes, you may have latent passions and talents that have not been explored yet. Allowing yourself to experience different and challenging activities can help you discover new interests and skills.

Exploring passions and talents often involves stepping out of your comfort zone. As you venture into new areas, you may encounter challenges and face uncertainty. However, it's in these moments of discomfort that growth occurs, and passions can flourish.

Consistent practice is necessary for developing talents.

Even if you have a natural inclination for something, practice and refinement are essential to reach your full potential.

Seeking guidance and learning is valuable. Finding mentors, teachers, or communities that share your interests can provide direction and support as you explore your passions and talents.

Sometimes, it can be helpful to think about what you would do if money were not a concern. This reflection can reveal deep passions you may have set aside due to financial considerations.

Patience is essential during this journey. Discovering and developing passions and talents often takes time, and it's normal to encounter obstacles along the way. The key is not to give up and continue persevering.

Self-awareness is an intrinsic part of this exploration. As you engage in activities that impassion you, you can learn more about your own values, motivations, and identity.

Overcoming the fear of judgment is important. Sometimes, we may hesitate to explore our passions and talents out of fear of what others will think. Self-confidence and authenticity are key to overcoming this obstacle.

Creating an environment that nurtures your passions and talents is crucial. This may involve organizing your time to allow for exploration, creating a dedicated space for your interests, or seeking out opportunities that connect you with people who share your passions.

The practice of gratitude plays an important role in this

journey. As you explore your passions and talents, it's important to recognize and appreciate the opportunities and resources that support you in your pursuit.

Authenticity is paramount. Sometimes, it can be tempting to pursue passions or talents that are popular or socially acceptable rather than following your own heart. However, finding and embracing what is authentically meaningful to you is essential for a satisfying life.

Exploring passions and talents often leads to a sense of purpose and meaning in life. When you engage in activities that impassion you, you are more likely to feel fulfilled and satisfied.

Building a support network is important. Having people who encourage and support you in your journey of exploring passions and talents can make all the difference.

Self-discovery is an ongoing process. As you evolve and grow, your passions and talents may change and expand. Being open to this evolution is important for continuous growth.

Exploring passions and talents is not just about the end result; it's also about the journey itself. The journey can be incredibly enriching and provide moments of joy and satisfaction.

In summary, exploring your passions and talents is a rewarding journey that involves self-reflection, willingness to try new things, stepping out of your comfort zone, consistent practice, seeking guidance, patience, self-awareness, and authenticity. It's a pursuit that can lead to a more meaningful life filled with purpose and satisfaction.

The Power of Self-Confidence: Believe in Yourself and Conquer Everything

3 DEVELOPING SELF-CONFIDENCE

Developing self-confidence is an exciting and transformative journey that empowers us to face challenges, pursue our goals, and live a more fulfilling and satisfying life. This chapter will delve deeply into this exploration, highlighting the essential steps to strengthen your self-confidence and build a solid foundation for success and well-being.

Self-confidence is not just a desirable quality but also a powerful tool that influences every aspect of our lives. It helps us make assertive decisions, face adversity with resilience, and cultivate healthy and meaningful relationships. Moreover, self-confidence empowers us to pursue our dreams with conviction, believe in our abilities, and overcome obstacles that might otherwise hold us back.

In this chapter, we will explore the roots of self-confidence, the obstacles that can undermine it, and the practical strategies that can be adopted to strengthen it. We will learn to transform self-criticism into self-compassion, confront fears and doubts, and cultivate a positive and resilient mindset. Most importantly, you will discover that self-confidence is a skill that can be developed and enhanced throughout life, empowering you to achieve your goals and live up to your true potential. So, prepare for a journey of self-discovery and growth as we explore the transformative power of self-confidence.

Strategies for Increasing Self-Confidence

Increasing self-confidence is an important pursuit that can significantly improve a person's quality of life. Self-confidence is not only a desirable personal trait but also a powerful tool for success in all aspects of life. Here, we will explore a variety of strategies to help strengthen your self-confidence and promote greater emotional well-being.

One of the most fundamental strategies for increasing self-confidence is self-reflection. This involves looking within yourself and assessing your abilities, achievements, and areas where you may feel less secure. Identifying your strengths and acknowledging your accomplishments can boost your self-esteem.

Challenging negative thoughts is crucial. We all have an inner critic that often makes us doubt our abilities and criticizes us relentlessly. Learning to identify and question these negative thoughts is an essential skill for building self-confidence.

Setting clear goals can be another effective strategy. Establishing clear and achievable goals can provide a clear direction and a sense of accomplishment as you reach them. Each small achievement contributes to strengthening self-confidence.

Practicing self-compassion is fundamental. Treating yourself with kindness and compassion, especially when you make mistakes or face challenges, is essential for a healthy self-image.

Accepting compliments and recognition is a skill that is often underestimated. When someone compliments you, accepting these compliments with gratitude rather than downplaying them can reinforce your self-esteem.

Stepping out of your comfort zone is a powerful strategy for increasing self-confidence. Facing challenges and trying new things, even if it is uncomfortable at first, can expand your limits and show you that you are capable of much more than you imagined.

Seeking guidance and support is important. Talking to friends, family, or a therapist can provide valuable external perspective and encouragement when you are working to increase your self-confidence.

Practicing assertiveness is a fundamental skill. Being able to express your needs, desires, and opinions respectfully and effectively helps build self-confidence and improves communication.

Positive visualization is a technique that can be used to boost self-confidence. Imagine yourself successfully performing a challenging task or achieving a specific goal. This mental practice can increase your confidence to face real situations.

Building a supportive environment is crucial. Surrounding yourself with people who encourage and believe in you is essential for strengthening self-confidence.

Continuous learning is an effective strategy. The more knowledge and skills you acquire, the more confident you will feel in your ability to face challenges.

Accepting that everyone makes mistakes is important. Not being too hard on yourself when something doesn't go as planned is an important aspect of building self-confidence.

Cultivating a positive mindset is essential. Replacing negative and constructive thoughts with positive ones can have a significant impact on self-confidence.

Seeking constructive feedback is valuable. Asking for feedback from colleagues or mentors can help identify areas for improvement and also highlight your achievements.

Creating an action plan is a practical strategy. Identifying specific steps to achieve a goal can provide a clear sense of direction and accomplishment.

Practicing gratitude plays an important role in building self-confidence. Recognizing and appreciating the good things in your life can improve your emotional well-being and boost self-esteem.

Establishing healthy boundaries is fundamental. Saying "no" when necessary and setting clear boundaries in relationships and obligations can help build self-confidence.

Taking care of your physical well-being is also important. Maintaining a balanced diet, regularly exercising, and getting adequate rest can improve self-image and self-confidence.

The practice of meditation and mindfulness is an effective way to calm the mind and reduce self-criticism, promoting a more positive self-image.

In summary, increasing self-confidence is a journey that involves self-reflection, challenging negative thoughts, setting goals, practicing self-compassion, accepting compliments, stepping out of your comfort zone, seeking guidance, practicing assertiveness, positive visualization, building a supportive environment, continuous learning, accepting mistakes, cultivating a positive mindset, seeking feedback, creating an action plan, practicing gratitude, establishing healthy boundaries, taking care of physical well-being, and meditation and mindfulness. By adopting these strategies, you can strengthen your self-confidence and face challenges with greater determination and success.

Overcoming Obstacles and Challenges

Overcoming obstacles and challenges is an inevitable part of life, and how we deal with them has a significant impact on our self-confidence and overall well-being. Although it can be difficult, facing these obstacles with resilience and determination can strengthen our self-confidence and help us grow as individuals.

One of the first steps in overcoming obstacles is adopting a positive mindset. Viewing challenges as opportunities for growth rather than insurmountable obstacles can dramatically change how we approach them. A positive mindset allows us to see obstacles as a natural part of life's journey.

Self-confidence plays a fundamental role in overcoming obstacles. When we believe in our own abilities and resilience, we are more willing to face challenges head-on and persevere when things get tough.

Developing resilience is a valuable skill. Resilience allows us to cope with adversity in an adaptive way and bounce back from failures or setbacks more easily. It also strengthens our self-confidence by showing us that we are capable of overcoming difficulties.

Setting clear goals can be an effective strategy for overcoming obstacles. When we have clear goals, we are more motivated to tackle challenges in order to achieve them. Achieving these goals strengthens our self-confidence.

Seeking social support is important. Talking to friends, family, or a therapist can provide emotional support and helpful perspectives when facing obstacles.

Practicing self-compassion is essential. Treating yourself with kindness and compassion, especially when facing difficulties, helps maintain a positive self-image.

Learning from experience is crucial. Every challenge we face offers learning opportunities. Reflecting on what you can learn from a tough situation can help you grow and build self-confidence.

Maintaining perspective is important. Sometimes, obstacles can seem overwhelming, but remembering that they are temporary and that you have overcome challenges in the past can provide strength and hope.

Patience plays a crucial role in overcoming obstacles. Not all problems are solved instantly, and it's important to be willing to persist and work gradually to overcome them.

Dealing with the fear of failure is a common challenge. Self-confidence is often undermined by the fear of not succeeding. It's important to recognize that failure is part of the path to success, and each failure is an opportunity for learning.

Creating an action plan is valuable. Identifying specific steps to address an obstacle or challenge can provide a sense of control and direction.

Seeking inspiring role models can motivate. Finding people who have overcome similar challenges can provide inspiration and show that overcoming obstacles is possible.

Problem-solving skills are a valuable skill. Developing the ability to analyze a problem, identify potential solutions, and implement the best strategy can help overcome obstacles more effectively.

Self-motivation plays a fundamental role. Sometimes, it's necessary to find internal motivation to face challenges and keep moving forward, even when things get tough.

Taking care of emotional well-being is important. Staying emotionally balanced and seeking support when needed can help overcome obstacles more effectively.

Accepting that not all obstacles can be avoided is fundamental. Some situations are beyond our control, and accepting this can alleviate the pressure of trying to avoid all challenges.

Seeking creative solutions is valuable. Sometimes, innovative thinking is required to overcome obstacles and find ways to work around problems.

The practice of persistence is essential. Continuing to work toward your goals, even when facing obstacles, is a crucial component of building self-confidence.

In summary, overcoming obstacles and challenges is a natural part of life, and how we face these situations can have a significant impact on our self-confidence and personal growth. Adopting a positive mindset, developing resilience, setting clear goals, seeking social support, and practicing self-compassion are some of the strategies that can help us overcome obstacles with more confidence and determination.

Learning from Experience

Learning from experience is a fundamental part of personal growth and the development of self-confidence. Every experience, whether positive or negative, offers valuable opportunities for learning and self-discovery. In this topic, we will explore how we can extract meaningful lessons from our experiences and use that knowledge to strengthen our self-confidence.

One of the first steps in learning from experience is reflection. This involves analyzing an experience, thinking about what happened, how you felt, and what the outcomes were. Reflection allows you to gain insights and better understand the situation.

Self-questioning is a powerful tool. Asking yourself questions like "What can I learn from this?" or "What could I have done differently?" helps guide your reflection and identify areas for growth.

The ability to find meaning in your experiences is important. Even in the most challenging situations, it is possible to find lessons and growth opportunities. This perspective can strengthen your resilience and self-confidence.

Seeking external feedback is valuable. Talking to others involved in an experience can provide different perspectives and insights that you may not have considered.

Accepting that making mistakes is part of the learning process is crucial. Often, we fear failure, but it's important to remember that making mistakes is an opportunity for growth. Self-confidence is strengthened when we realize that failure does not define us.

Self-compassion plays a fundamental role in learning from experience. Treating yourself with kindness and compassion, especially when you make mistakes, is essential for maintaining a healthy self-image.

The practice of adaptation is important. As you learn from your experiences, it's crucial to apply the knowledge gained to make more informed decisions in the future.

Keeping a journal or taking notes about your experiences can be helpful. This allows you to track your learning process and reflect on changes over time.

Seeking inspiring role models can motivate. Finding people who have gone through similar experiences and successfully overcome them can provide guidance and inspiration.

Building a growth mindset is essential. Believing that your intelligence and abilities can be developed over time promotes a willingness to learn from experiences.

Practicing empathy is important when learning from interactive experiences. Putting yourself in the shoes of others involved in a situation can help you better understand the dynamics and feelings involved.

Seeking opportunities for continuous learning is valuable. Each new experience offers a chance to acquire new knowledge and skills, thereby strengthening self-confidence.

Building resilience is a natural outcome of learning from experience. The more you face challenges and overcome obstacles, the more confident you become in your ability to handle difficult situations.

Sharing your own experiences can benefit others. Sometimes, by sharing your learned lessons, you can inspire and help others in their own learning journeys.

Accepting that not all experiences are positive is important. It is natural to go through tough times, and these experiences can shape your resilience and self-confidence.

The practice of gratitude plays an important role in appreciating life's lessons. Recognizing and being grateful for learning opportunities can improve your emotional well-being.

Creating an environment that encourages learning is crucial. Surrounding yourself with people who value learning and personal growth can motivate you to learn from your experiences.

Seeking new experiences is an effective way to expand your knowledge and perspectives. Stepping out of your comfort zone and exposing yourself to different situations can enrich your life and your confidence.

Continuous self-assessment is an important practice. As you learn from your experiences, it's important to regularly evaluate your progress and adjust your actions as needed.

In summary, learning from experience is a valuable skill that can strengthen your self-confidence and promote significant personal growth. Reflection, self-questioning, seeking feedback, accepting mistakes, and applying acquired knowledge are some of the essential elements of this journey of continuous learning.

4 DEALING WITH SELF-REALIZATION

Dealing with self-realization is a profound journey in search of our maximum potential and the fulfillment of our most significant goals. This chapter will lead us to explore the meaning of self-realization and the strategies to achieve it. It is an exploration that invites us to reflect on who we are, what we wish to achieve, and how we can make our dreams and aspirations a reality.

Self-realization is a concept that goes beyond the simple pursuit of material success; it is about achieving a state of fulfillment and personal satisfaction. It is the realization of our values, passions, and life purpose. It involves the journey of discovering our true passions, talents, and goals, and then actively working to manifest them in our lives.

In this chapter, we will explore the different dimensions of self-realization, including personal development, the search for meaning, creativity, and contributing to the well-being of society. We will discuss how to identify our passions, overcome obstacles, and create an action plan to get closer to our deepest goals.

Furthermore, we will explore the importance of authenticity and self-connection along this path. Self-realization involves living in alignment with our deepest values and beliefs, finding the true expression of who we are.

As we delve into this journey of self-realization, I invite you to open yourself to the possibility of growth and transformation. Throughout this chapter, we will discover that self-realization is not just a destination but a continuous journey of self-discovery and evolution. Therefore, prepare to explore the unlimited potential that exists within you and take significant steps toward the full realization of your life.

Setting Goals and Objectives

Setting goals and objectives is a fundamental step in the journey of self-realization. This implies not only understanding what we want to achieve but also establishing a clear plan to get there. In this topic, we will explore the importance of setting goals and objectives and how it contributes to our pursuit of self-realization.

Goals and objectives provide a sense of direction. They give us purpose and focus for our daily actions. When we have clear goals in mind, we know where we are going and why we are doing what we do. This can help us avoid feeling adrift in life.

Moreover, goals challenge us to grow. When we set goals that are beyond our current abilities, we are encouraged to learn, improve, and expand our capabilities.

This directly contributes to personal development, a crucial component of self-realization.

Goals also help us measure progress. By setting measurable milestones and objectives, we can track our advancement over time. This allows us to celebrate our achievements and adjust our course if necessary.

Defining goals and objectives helps us overcome procrastination. When we have a goal in mind, we are more likely to take immediate action to achieve it. This prevents us from postponing our dreams and aspirations.

Goals and objectives can be a source of motivation. They provide us with a reason to strive and keep us energized and committed to our pursuit of self-realization.

However, it is important that goals are meaningful and aligned with our values and passions. Setting goals that lack profound meaning for us can lead to a sense of emptiness and unfulfillment, even if they are achieved.

It is crucial to set realistic and achievable goals. Establishing goals that are beyond our abilities or current resources can lead to frustration and discouragement. Finding a balance between challenging and attainable goals is important.

Additionally, it is valuable to set short-term, medium-term, and long-term goals. This allows us to have a comprehensive plan and break our journey into manageable steps. Short-term goals can provide us with a sense of immediate achievement, while long-term goals give us a vision of the future.

Flexibility is important when setting goals. Sometimes, life presents unexpected changes and challenges that may require us to adapt our objectives. Being open to adjusting our goals as our journey of self-realization evolves is essential.

Visualization is a powerful technique that can be used when setting goals. Imagine yourself successfully achieving your goals; visualize how you will feel when you attain them. This can increase your motivation and make your goals more tangible.

Planning is essential. Creating a detailed action plan that includes the necessary steps to reach your goals can provide a clear roadmap for achievement.

Seeking support and guidance is valuable. Sometimes, sharing your goals with friends, family, or mentors can provide emotional support and helpful advice.

In summary, setting goals and objectives is a fundamental part of the pursuit of self-realization. They provide direction, challenge, motivation, and a way to measure our progress. However, it is important that these goals are meaningful, realistic, and aligned with our values and passions. By embracing goal setting as part of your self-realization journey, you are taking a significant step toward realizing your full potential.

Persevering in Pursuit of Your Dreams

Persevering in the pursuit of your dreams is a crucial skill on the path of self-realization. Often, the most significant goals require time, effort, and facing significant challenges. In this topic, we will explore the importance of perseverance and how you can cultivate this quality to achieve your deepest dreams.

One of the first lessons in perseverance is understanding that success rarely happens overnight. The journey toward your dreams can be filled with ups and downs, and it is essential to be prepared to overcome the obstacles that arise.

Maintaining focus on your goals is essential. Sometimes, distractions and adversities can divert our attention, but perseverance involves the ability to keep your vision clear and keep moving forward, even when the journey becomes challenging.

Resilience plays a crucial role in perseverance. It is the ability to bounce back from setbacks, learn from failures, and continue moving forward with determination. Resilience is one of the pillars of self-realization as it allows you to overcome adversity.

Self-confidence is a motivating factor in perseverance. When you believe in your abilities and the possibility of achieving your dreams, you are more willing to face challenges with confidence.

Setting clear goals can aid in perseverance. When you have specific objectives in mind, you are more motivated to overcome the obstacles that arise along the way.

Adaptation is a valuable skill in the pursuit of dreams. Sometimes, it is necessary to adjust your approach or strategy as you encounter new challenges or unforeseen circumstances.

Patience is a virtue when it comes to perseverance. You may not always see immediate results, and it is important to be willing to keep working toward your dreams, even when results take time.

Creating a detailed action plan is crucial. Having a clear roadmap that includes steps and measurable goals can help you stay on track and provide a sense of direction.

Maintaining a positive mindset is important in the pursuit of your dreams. Cultivating optimism and believing that you can overcome challenges contributes to perseverance.

Seeking support is valuable. Sharing your dreams and challenges with friends, family, or mentors can provide emotional support and helpful guidance.

Self-motivation plays a fundamental role in perseverance. Finding internal motivation to keep moving forward, even when things get tough, is important.

Dealing with the fear of failure is a common challenge in the pursuit of dreams. Self-confidence and resilience play an important role in overcoming this fear, allowing you to keep moving forward despite doubts.

Celebrating small victories is important. As you work toward your dreams, it is essential to recognize and celebrate each achievement, no matter how small it may seem.

Seeking inspiring role models can motivate. Finding people who have achieved similar success to what you aspire to can provide inspiration and guidance along the way.

Self-motivation plays a fundamental role in perseverance. Finding internal motivation to keep moving forward, even when things get tough, is important.

Seeking support is valuable. Sharing your dreams and challenges with friends, family, or mentors can provide emotional support and helpful guidance.

Creating an environment that encourages perseverance is crucial. Surrounding yourself with people who believe in your dreams and encourage you to keep going is essential.

Accepting that the journey of self-realization can be challenging but rewarding is important. It is normal to encounter difficulties along the way, but perseverance will take you there.

In summary, persevering in the pursuit of your dreams is a vital quality on the journey of self-realization. It requires resilience, self-confidence, determination, and a continuous commitment to your goals. By embracing perseverance, you come closer to the fulfillment of your deepest dreams and experience personal growth along the way.

Celebrating Personal Achievements

Celebrating personal achievements is an essential part of the journey of self-realization. Often, we are so focused on achieving our goals that we forget to recognize and celebrate the milestones along the way. In this topic, we will explore the importance of celebrating personal achievements and how this practice can strengthen our self-confidence and well-being.

One of the main reasons for celebrating personal achievements is that it allows us to acknowledge and appreciate our own progress. Often, we are our harshest critics and tend to downplay our accomplishments. By pausing and celebrating, we give ourselves the validation we deserve.

Celebrating personal achievements creates a positive cycle of reinforcement. When we recognize and celebrate our successes, we release dopamine, the pleasure neurotransmitter, which makes us feel good and motivates us to keep progressing.

Furthermore, celebrating personal achievements boosts our self-confidence. When we remember and celebrate the times, we overcame challenges or achieved goals, our belief in our own abilities and capabilities increases.

Celebration also allows us to have a more balanced perspective. Sometimes, we become so focused on what we have not yet achieved that we forget how much we have already accomplished. This can lead to feelings of dissatisfaction and discouragement.

It is important that the celebration is personalized and meaningful to you. It can range from small personal rituals, such as taking time for reflection and gratitude, to more elaborate celebrations with friends and family.

When celebrating personal achievements, it is valuable to express gratitude to yourself. Acknowledge the effort, determination, and resilience you have shown in reaching your goals.

Celebration is also an opportunity to reflect on progress
and future challenges. Use this moment to consider what
you have learned on your journey and how you can apply
those lessons to your next steps.

Celebrating personal achievements with others can
strengthen social bonds. Sharing your joys and
accomplishments with friends and family creates deeper
connections and strengthens relationships.

Remembering your past achievements can serve as a
source of motivation. When facing new challenges or
difficult moments, thinking about the times you overcame
obstacles in the past can give you the confidence needed to
persevere.

Celebration is also a way to create special moments and
meaningful memories. When we look back on our lives, we
remember not only the goals we achieved but also the
experiences and emotions associated with those moments
of celebration.

It is important to remember that all personal
achievements, no matter how small or large, deserve to be
celebrated. From professional accomplishments to personal
milestones, every step toward self-realization is significant.

Celebration does not need to be extravagant or costly.
Sometimes, the most meaningful celebrations are simple
and authentic, such as taking a moment to savor a cup of
coffee while reflecting on a personal achievement.

Celebration is also a way to express self-worth. When

you acknowledge and celebrate your achievements, you are
sending yourself the message that you deserve recognition
and care.

In summary, celebrating personal achievements is an
important practice on the journey of self-realization. It
helps us recognize our progress, reinforces our self-
confidence, creates a positive cycle of reinforcement, and
allows us to value our own efforts. By incorporating
celebration into your life, you not only enrich your journey
of self-realization but also find joy and gratitude along the
way.

5 SELF-CONFIDENCE IN INTERPERSONAL RELATIONSHIPS

This chapter takes us on a fascinating journey through the universe of human connections and how self-confidence plays a fundamental role in our relationships. As we explore this topic, we will unravel how believing in oneself can positively influence the way we connect with others and build meaningful relationships.

Interpersonal relationships are an integral part of our daily life, from friendships and family relationships to professional and romantic partnerships. As social beings, we seek meaningful connections with others, and the quality of these connections is often intrinsically linked to our self-confidence.

Self-confidence in relationships is not just about feeling good about oneself but also about how it affects our ability to communicate, establish healthy boundaries, express our needs, and deal with conflicts constructively. Therefore, this chapter invites us to explore how we can cultivate self-confidence to create more fulfilling and meaningful relationships.

In the pages that follow, we will delve into topics such as the importance of effective communication, building healthy relationships, and overcoming challenges in interpersonal interactions. We will explore how self-confidence not only strengthens our ability to create positive connections but also helps us cope with rejection, criticism, and navigate challenging social situations.

Additionally, we will examine how self-confidence can play a fundamental role in our ability to set healthy boundaries, make assertive decisions, and maintain balanced relationships. Through real-life examples and practical strategies, this chapter will provide valuable insights into how you can strengthen your self-confidence and improve your interpersonal relationships.

I invite you to explore this chapter with an open mind and a receptive heart. By doing so, you will be on the path to enhancing your relationship skills, building deeper bonds with others, and experiencing a more satisfying and harmonious social life. Self-confidence is a powerful tool, and this chapter is your guide to using it to create more meaningful and enriching interpersonal connections.

Building Healthy Relationships

Building healthy relationships is a vital skill on the journey of self-confidence in interpersonal relationships. These relationships are the foundation of a rewarding social life and play a crucial role in our emotional and mental well-being. In this topic, we will explore how we can build healthy relationships, strengthen our self-confidence, and contribute to mutual growth and happiness.

First and foremost, it is essential to have clarity about who we are and what we value in a relationship. This involves knowing our own limits, needs, and desires. When we have a solid understanding of ourselves, we can establish a strong foundation for healthy relationships.

Communication plays a central role in building healthy relationships. This includes the ability to express our feelings, thoughts, and needs openly and honestly. Self-confidence plays a crucial role here as it enables us to communicate our feelings and needs assertively.

Mutual respect is a fundamental pillar of any healthy relationship. This means honoring each other's individuality, opinions, and boundaries. Self-confidence allows us to maintain our self-respect and dignity while also showing respect for others.

Empathy is a valuable quality in building healthy relationships. Putting oneself in the other person's shoes, understanding their emotions and perspectives, and demonstrating compassion contribute to emotional connection.

Trust is a crucial part of healthy relationships. Self-confidence is the foundation for trusting others and, at the same time, trusting ourselves to make decisions and face challenges together.

Setting healthy boundaries is important in building relationships. This involves clearly communicating our personal boundaries and respecting the boundaries of others. Self-confidence enables us to establish and maintain these boundaries firmly and respectfully.

Conflict resolution is an essential skill. All relationships face challenges and disagreements from time to time. Self-confidence gives us the courage to address conflicts constructively, seeking solutions that benefit both parties.

Pursuing common interests and shared goals strengthens healthy relationships. This creates a sense of purpose and collaboration, which can be very rewarding and motivating.

Flexibility is important in building healthy relationships. As life evolves, our relationships also need to adapt. Self-confidence helps us face changes and uncertainties with resilience.

Reciprocity is a key element in healthy relationships. This means that both you and your partner are willing to give and receive support, love, and care in a balanced manner.

Building healthy relationships requires patience and time investment. It is not something that happens overnight but rather a continuous journey of growth and deepening connections.

Celebrating moments and achievements together is a way to nurture healthy relationships. Celebrating milestones and sharing moments of joy creates stronger bonds.

In summary, building healthy relationships is a complex process that involves self-awareness, effective communication, mutual respect, empathy, trust, and much more. Self-confidence plays a vital role in this process, allowing you to relate to others authentically and assertively. When we cultivate healthy relationships, we contribute to our own well-being and the well-being of those around us.

Communicating with Confidence

Communicating with confidence is a valuable skill that impacts all areas of our lives, from personal relationships to career and goal achievement. Confidence in communication not only helps us convey our ideas more effectively but also influences how others perceive us. In this topic, we will explore the importance of communicating with confidence and how developing this skill can strengthen our self-confidence.

Communication is a fundamental part of our daily interactions. It includes not only what we say but also how we say it, our body language, facial expressions, and tone of voice. Effective communication involves the ability to convey our messages clearly and assertively.

Confidence in communication starts with confidence in oneself. When we believe in our ideas, opinions, and knowledge, our communication reflects that self-confidence. This influences how we express our ideas and how we defend them.

Confident communication also involves the ability to listen attentively. Self-confidence allows us to listen without feeling the constant need to interrupt or feel insecure about what others are saying.

Self-confidence in communication helps us handle

challenges such as negotiations, conflicts, and public speaking. Believing in our ability to face these situations enables us to approach them calmly and assertively.

Body language plays a significant role in confident communication. Upright posture, eye contact, and confident gestures are indicators of confidence and impact how we are perceived by others.

Self-confidence in communication is also linked to empathy. When we communicate with empathy, we show consideration for others' feelings and perspectives, creating healthier and more productive relationships.

Authenticity is a fundamental component of confident communication. Being authentic means being true to oneself and expressing thoughts and feelings honestly.

Confidence in communication influences our ability to build solid and trustworthy relationships. Trust is a fundamental foundation for healthy relationships, and effective communication is a means of building that trust.

Communicating with confidence does not mean being arrogant or domineering. It's about expressing your ideas and opinions with respect for others and openness to dialogue.

Confident communication is a skill that can be learned and improved over time. This involves practicing assertive communication, developing listening skills, and being aware of your body language.

Self-assessment is a valuable tool for developing confident communication. This involves reflecting on your own communication, identifying areas for improvement, and working on them consistently.

Self-confidence in communication is not limited to speaking; it also relates to writing. The ability to express your ideas clearly and persuasively in writing is a valuable skill in many contexts.

Dealing with the fear of judgment from others is a common challenge in communication. Self-confidence helps us confront this fear and communicate our ideas even when there is a possibility of disagreement.

In summary, communicating with confidence is a vital skill that influences how we interact with the world. Confidence in communication helps us express our ideas effectively, build healthy relationships, and address communication challenges calmly and assertively. Cultivating this skill not only strengthens our self-confidence but also improves our ability to positively influence others and achieve our goals. This topic is a guide to developing confident communication as a powerful tool for success and fulfillment in all areas of your life.

Dealing with Conflicts Positively

Dealing with conflicts positively is a fundamental skill in any interpersonal relationship. Conflicts are inevitable in our lives, but how we approach and resolve them can make the difference between creating resentment and strengthening bonds. In this topic, we will explore strategies and approaches for addressing conflicts constructively while maintaining self-confidence and integrity in relationships.

First and foremost, it's important to acknowledge that conflicts are normal and part of the human experience. They can arise due to differences of opinion, unmet expectations, misunderstandings, or unfulfilled needs. Self-confidence provides the foundation for facing conflicts calmly and courageously, rather than avoiding or suppressing them.

Communication is key to dealing with conflicts positively. This involves clearly expressing your feelings and concerns in a respectful manner and actively listening to the other person's point of view. Self-confidence plays an important role in the ability to communicate your needs and emotions assertively.

Practicing empathy is valuable when dealing with conflicts. Try to understand the other person's perspective and acknowledge their emotions and concerns. This can create an atmosphere of mutual understanding.

Keeping calm during a conflict is essential. Self-confidence can help you remain composed and in control even when emotions are running high. This allows you to think more clearly and make thoughtful decisions.

Seeking solutions together is an important goal in conflict resolution. Instead of focusing on blame or winning, work with the other person to find mutually beneficial ways to resolve the issue.

Negotiation plays a crucial role in conflict resolution. This involves compromise and flexibility as both parties give in some areas to reach a satisfactory agreement.

Setting healthy boundaries during a conflict is important.

This involves maintaining mutual respect, avoiding personal attacks, and ensuring that communication remains constructive.

Learning from conflicts is a valuable opportunity. Conflicts can reveal areas where communication or understanding is weak and offer a chance to improve those areas.

Self-reflection after a conflict is helpful. Ask yourself what you've learned and how you can avoid similar conflicts in the future.

Forgiveness is an important part of conflict resolution. Forgiving doesn't necessarily mean forgetting, but rather letting go of resentment and moving forward.

Avoiding the use of hurtful language or accusations during a conflict is crucial. Self-confidence can help you maintain respectful communication even when emotions are high.

Sometimes, seeking the guidance of a mediator or impartial third party can help resolve a conflict.

The importance of keeping a common goal in mind during a conflict cannot be underestimated. This helps maintain focus on problem resolution rather than clinging to resentments or past arguments.

Self-confidence plays a crucial role in the ability to face and resolve conflicts positively. It gives you the security to express your needs and concerns and the courage to address interpersonal challenges with respect and empathy. By embracing conflict resolution as an opportunity for personal growth and relationship enhancement, you strengthen your connections and contribute to a more harmonious environment in your life.

6 SELF-CONFIDENCE IN WORK AND CAREER

This chapter takes us on an exciting exploration of the complexities of self-confidence in the professional context. In the workplace, self-confidence plays a vital role in our ability to succeed, grow, and thrive. As we delve into this topic, we will discover how believing in oneself can shape our career and influence our professional journey.

The workplace is a dynamic and challenging setting where opportunities intertwine with challenges. Self-confidence is a powerful tool that helps us confront these challenges with resilience and determination. In this chapter, we will explore how self-confidence can affect our ability to take on new responsibilities, face challenges, lead teams, and seek growth opportunities.

Furthermore, we will examine how self-confidence plays a fundamental role in how we present ourselves in the workplace. It influences how we communicate, how we position ourselves, and how we interact with colleagues, superiors, and subordinates. Self-confidence is a quality that can attract opportunities and inspire confidence in those around us.

Striking a balance between challenging oneself and avoiding self-sabotage is an ongoing journey. Self-confidence gives us the courage to pursue new challenges, even if it involves risks, and also prevents us from underestimating our own skills and contributions.

In this chapter, we will explore how self-confidence is a key piece of the puzzle for professional satisfaction and success. We will examine practical strategies to strengthen your self-confidence at work, overcome specific challenges in the professional environment, and build a solid and rewarding career.

I invite you to explore this chapter with an open mind and a critical look at your own self-confidence at work. By doing so, you will be on the path to maximizing your professional potential, achieving your career goals, and successfully navigating the complex world of work and career. Self-confidence is a skill that can be developed and enhanced, and this chapter is your guide to mastering it in the professional context.

Excelling in the Professional Environment

Excelling in the professional environment is a goal cherished by many, and self-confidence plays a central role in the pursuit of success and recognition. In this topic, we will explore how cultivating self-confidence can help you stand out and thrive in your career, regardless of the industry or hierarchical level.

The Power of Self-Confidence: Believe in Yourself and Conquer
Everything

Self-confidence is a quality that attracts attention and inspires confidence in others. When you believe in yourself, others are more likely to believe in you as well. This perceived confidence can open doors to leadership opportunities and collaborations.

A positive self-image and self-esteem are essential components of self-confidence. When you value yourself and acknowledge your own skills and achievements, it is reflected in your attitude and behavior in the workplace. People are naturally drawn to individuals who are comfortable with themselves.

Self-confidence also influences how you deal with challenges and adversities at work. Instead of being seen as insurmountable obstacles, challenges are viewed as opportunities for growth and learning. Self-confidence gives you the resilience to overcome setbacks and keep moving forward.

The ability to take calculated risks is another advantage of self-confidence in the professional environment. In many cases, success requires a willingness to step out of your comfort zone and face the unknown. Confidence in your abilities and judgment can make these decisions easier to make.

Self-confidence also manifests in effective communication. When you believe in yourself, you are better able to express your ideas clearly and assertively. This is crucial in meetings, presentations, and interactions with colleagues and superiors.

Leadership is a domain where self-confidence is

particularly valuable. Self-confident leaders inspire their teams, provide direction, and face challenges with courage. Self-confidence also helps leaders make tough decisions and take responsibility for their outcomes.

Self-confidence is closely linked to the ability to establish solid professional relationships. Confidence in yourself allows you to build authentic connections with colleagues, superiors, and subordinates, contributing to a collaborative and harmonious work environment.

Developing self-confidence in the professional environment involves authenticity. This means being true to yourself and not trying to be someone you're not to please others. Authenticity is valued and creates genuine relationships.

Self-confidence is not static; it can be cultivated and improved over time. This requires self-awareness, self-reflection, and continuous self-development. By recognizing your weaknesses and working to improve them, you strengthen your self-confidence.

It's important to remember that self-confidence is not arrogance. Being self-confident does not mean underestimating others or ignoring their contributions. On the contrary, it involves recognizing and valuing the skills and perspectives of everyone.

In summary, excelling in the professional environment is intrinsically linked to your self-confidence. It shapes your image, influences your approach to challenges, affects your communication, and plays a vital role in your leadership and career growth journey. Cultivating self-confidence is a skill that can open doors, inspire confidence, and help you achieve your professional goals. This chapter is a guide to strengthening your self-confidence and harnessing it to the fullest in the workplace.

Leadership and Self-Confidence

Leadership and self-confidence are intrinsically linked. Effective leadership often requires a strong foundation of self-confidence, as leaders need to make tough decisions, face challenges, and inspire their teams. In this topic, we will explore the relationship between leadership and self-confidence, highlighting how believing in oneself can make you a more effective leader.

A self-confident leader inspires confidence in their team. When you demonstrate confidence in your own abilities and in your team's capabilities, it creates a more positive and productive work environment. Team members feel secure and motivated under the leadership of someone who believes in themselves.

Self-confidence enables leaders to make decisive decisions. Leaders often need to choose the most appropriate course of action for the team and the organization, which may involve risks. Confidence in your decision-making abilities helps you make assertive choices.

Self-confident leaders are more likely to take responsibility for their results. They don't seek blame but rather solutions. This creates an environment of accountability and respect, where team members feel valued and supported.

Self-confidence also plays a crucial role in

communication. Leaders need to express their visions, goals, and expectations clearly and convincingly. The ability to communicate effectively helps keep the team aligned and motivated.

Authenticity is valued in leadership. Leaders who are authentic and show who they truly are inspire confidence and connection. Self-confidence allows you to be more authentic and truer to yourself as a leader.

Self-confident leaders are more resilient. They can face adversity and challenges with courage and determination. This creates an environment where the team also becomes more resilient.

Self-confidence is a fundamental part of a leader's charisma. Charisma is the ability to attract and influence others, and self-confidence plays an important role in this aspect. Self-confident leaders have a magnetic presence that draws others to follow them.

Self-confidence also helps leaders establish healthy boundaries. This means they can set clear expectations for the team and ensure everyone is working toward common goals.

Developing self-confidence as a leader involves self-awareness and continuous self-improvement. This may include seeking constructive feedback, developing new skills, and managing workplace stress and pressure.

Humility is also important in leadership. Self-confidence should not be confused with arrogance. Self-confident leaders acknowledge their own shortcomings and are willing to learn from others.

Self-confidence is contagious. When a leader believes in themselves, it inspires team members to believe in themselves and their work.

In summary, leadership and self-confidence are closely related. Believing in oneself as a leader is not just an advantage but an essential quality. Self-confidence influences how you lead, make decisions, communicate with your team, and face challenges. Cultivating self-confidence as a leader is an ongoing journey that can lead to more effective performance and personal as well as professional growth. This chapter is a guide to strengthening your self-confidence and using it to become a more effective and influential leader.

Achieving Professional Success

Achieving professional success is a goal that many aspire to, and self-confidence plays a fundamental role in this process. Professional success is not just about achieving financial goals or attaining a prestigious position, but also about experiencing personal fulfillment and satisfaction in your career. In this topic, we will explore how believing in yourself can drive your ambitions and help you achieve the professional success you desire.

Self-confidence influences how you set professional goals. Self-confident individuals are more likely to set ambitious goals and believe they can achieve them. This motivates them to consistently work towards these goals.

Self-confidence helps overcome obstacles in the pursuit of success. In any career, there will be challenges and setbacks. Self-confidence strengthens your resilience, enabling you to face these obstacles with determination and adaptability.

It also influences your ability to take calculated risks. Success often requires the willingness to step out of your comfort zone and explore new opportunities. Self-confidence gives you the courage to confront these challenges with confidence in your skills and judgment.

Self-confidence is also a significant factor in seeking career advancement opportunities. When you believe in yourself, you are more likely to pursue promotions, new projects, and additional responsibilities that can propel your career forward.

Communication is essential for professional success, and self-confidence plays a vital role here. Self-confident individuals are better able to express themselves clearly and assertively, which is valued in the workplace.

Self-confidence influences how you present yourself at work. It helps build a positive professional image, which can increase your chances of being noticed and recognized for your achievements.

The pursuit of learning and development opportunities is a common trait among self-confident individuals. They recognize that professional success often requires continuous skill and knowledge enhancement.

Self-confidence also affects how you handle feedback. Instead of viewing feedback as personal criticism, self-confident individuals use it as an opportunity for learning and growth.

Managing stress and pressure at work is crucial for professional success. Self-confidence helps you stay calm and make thoughtful decisions, even in challenging situations.

Building strong professional relationships is also critical for success. Self-confident individuals are better able to establish authentic and constructive connections with colleagues, superiors, and clients.

Striking a balance between work and personal life is an important aspect of success. Self-confidence helps you establish healthy boundaries and prioritize your personal needs, contributing to a balanced and successful life.

It's important to remember that professional success is not a linear journey, and there will be ups and downs along the way. Self-confidence gives you the strength to persist and continue pursuing your goals, even in the face of challenges. Self-confidence is also linked to resilience. Self-confident individuals are better able to quickly recover from failures and keep moving towards success.

In summary, achieving professional success requires self-confidence. It influences your ability to set ambitious goals, face challenges, take risks, communicate effectively, and build strong professional relationships. Cultivating and strengthening self-confidence is an ongoing journey that can lead to significant achievements in your career. This chapter is a guide to developing your self-confidence and using it as a powerful tool to achieve the professional success you desire.

7 MAINTAINING SELF-CONFIDENCE THROUGHOUT LIFE

This chapter takes us on a journey of reflection and self-discovery about the importance of self-confidence at every stage of our lives. Self-confidence is not a quality we acquire once and maintain forever; it is a skill that needs to be cultivated and nurtured over time. In this chapter, we will explore how we can maintain and strengthen our self-confidence as we face the challenges and changes that life presents to us.

Throughout life, we are confronted with various transitions and obstacles, whether in our careers, relationships, health, or self-esteem. Maintaining strong self-confidence becomes essential for facing these changes with resilience and determination. As we explore this topic, we will examine strategies and approaches to preserve and reinforce our self-confidence at every stage of the journey.

From childhood to old age, self-confidence plays a vital role in how we face challenges, seek opportunities, and relate to others. Throughout this chapter, we will highlight how self-confidence can help us stay motivated, make informed decisions, and handle the ups and downs that life throws our way.

I invite you to explore this chapter with an open mind and a willingness for continuous self-development. Regardless of your age or life stage, self-confidence is a skill that can be cultivated and enhanced, and this chapter is a guide to keeping it strong and resilient throughout your entire journey. As we progress, we will discover how self-confidence is a constant ally in our pursuit of a fulfilling and meaningful life.

Overcoming Challenges and Changes

Overcoming challenges and changes is an inevitable part of every individual's life journey. The ability to face these obstacles with self-confidence plays a crucial role in how we navigate the complexities of existence. In this topic, we will explore the importance of self-confidence in overcoming challenges and adapting to changes, regardless of their nature or magnitude.

Challenges can take many forms, from personal adversities such as health issues or losses to professional, academic, or social challenges. Regardless of the type of challenge we face, our self-confidence significantly influences our response to these situations.

Self-confidence helps us stay calm under pressure. When we encounter challenges, emotions like fear and anxiety often arise. Self-confidence provides us with emotional resilience to face these feelings and make thoughtful decisions.

Furthermore, self-confidence gives us the courage to confront challenges head-on instead of avoiding them. Believing in our own abilities encourages us to seek solutions and proactively address problems.

Self-confidence is also linked to resilience. It helps us recover from setbacks and view challenges as opportunities for growth. Rather than being discouraged by difficulties, self-confidence motivates us to learn from them and move forward.

Self-confidence is particularly valuable in times of change. When facing significant life transitions such as job changes, relocations, divorce, or the loss of loved ones, self-confidence helps us cope with uncertainty and adapt to new circumstances.

It also influences our ability to make informed decisions during times of change. By believing in our ability to make wise decisions and evaluate available options, we can approach changes with confidence.

Self-confidence is essential for dealing with self-criticism and perfectionism. Often, we are our harshest critics. Self-confidence helps us combat these negative patterns and maintain a more positive and constructive self-view.

When facing challenges and changes, self-confidence also influences how we seek support and resources. Self-confident individuals are more likely to seek help when needed and build strong support networks.

Maintaining self-confidence during difficult times can be

challenging, but it is a valuable skill. This involves practicing self-reflection and remembering your past achievements and strengths, even when things are tough.

Emotional resilience is also an important aspect of self-confidence. It means being able to regulate your emotions and cope with stress in a healthy way.

Self-compassion is a quality related to self-confidence. It is the ability to treat oneself with kindness and understanding, even when making mistakes or facing challenges.

In summary, overcoming challenges and changes in life requires self-confidence. It shapes our emotional response, our ability to confront problems head-on, our resilience, and our adaptability to change. Cultivating and strengthening self-confidence is a valuable investment for facing the challenges and uncertainties that life inevitably presents. This chapter is a guide to developing and maintaining your self-confidence in the face of life's complexities with courage and determination.

The Importance of Self-Care

The importance of self-care transcends all areas of our lives, from physical and mental health to emotional and spiritual well-being. It is a fundamental pillar for keeping self-confidence high and facing life's challenges with resilience. In this topic, we will explore the essential nature of self-care, highlighting how investing in oneself can be a powerful foundation for strengthening and preserving self-confidence.

Self-care involves dedicating time and energy to taking care of our physical, emotional, and mental needs. This includes habits like healthy eating, regular exercise, quality sleep, and attention to physical health.

Maintaining good mental health is equally vital. This involves practices such as stress management, meditation, therapy, or other activities that promote emotional balance.

Self-care is not limited to the body and mind; it also extends to our environment and lifestyle. This involves creating a living space that fosters peace and comfort, as well as setting healthy boundaries regarding work and obligations.

Self-confidence is often linked to self-esteem. Taking care of oneself nurtures self-esteem, as you acknowledge that you are worthy of attention and care. High self-esteem is a solid foundation for self-confidence.

Moreover, self-care also influences how we handle challenges and adversities. When we are well-cared for, we are more resilient and capable of facing obstacles with a positive mindset.

Self-care is a form of self-commitment. It means prioritizing your own needs, not as an act of selfishness but as a recognition that by taking care of yourself, you become better equipped to care for others.

Often, the lack of self-care can lead to physical and emotional burnout. This, in turn, can undermine self-confidence, making it more challenging to deal with challenges and make assertive decisions.

It's important to emphasize that self-care is not a luxury; it is a fundamental need for a balanced and healthy life. Neglecting self-care can have negative consequences for long-term health and well-being.

The consistent practice of self-care creates a positive cycle. When you take care of yourself, you feel better about yourself, which strengthens self-confidence. Self-confidence, in turn, fuels the desire to continue investing in your own well-being.

Self-care is also related to the ability to set healthy boundaries. This means saying no when necessary and not overwhelming yourself with obligations that harm your health and well-being.

Self-care is not a static concept; it evolves over time and circumstances. What you need for self-care can change, and it's important to adjust your self-care practices according to your evolving needs.

In summary, the importance of self-care in maintaining self-confidence is undeniable. It nurtures our physical and mental health, strengthens our self-esteem, enhances our resilience, and helps us face challenges with a positive mindset. Cultivating self-care is not an act of selfishness but an act of self-love and a wise choice that benefits not only you but also those around you. This chapter is a guide to incorporating self-care into your life as a constant ally on the journey of self-confidence and lasting well-being.

Drawing Inspiration and Inspiring Others

Drawing inspiration and inspiring others is a virtuous

cycle that plays a fundamental role in building and maintaining self-confidence. When we seek inspiration, we find motivation and encouragement to pursue our goals and overcome challenges. At the same time, when we inspire others, we strengthen our own self-confidence because we realize the positive impact, we can have on the lives of people around us. In this topic, we will explore the importance of this process of mutual inspiration and how it contributes to our self-confidence.

Inspiration often arises from models or figures we admire. By observing the achievements and challenges overcome by other people, we are motivated to pursue our own goals and overcome our obstacles.

The search for inspiration is a form of self-reflection. We question our values, goals, and aspirations when we feel inspired by someone or something. This helps strengthen our self-confidence as it helps us understand what is important to us and creates a sense of purpose.

Inspiring others is a manifestation of self-confidence because it requires us to share our own experiences and wisdom. When we can inspire someone, it validates our own journeys and achievements, strengthening our self-confidence.

Inspiration is a way to build meaningful relationships. When we inspire or are inspired by others, it creates authentic connections and shared experiences, which are vital for our self-confidence.

Inspiring others is also a way to contribute to the well-being of the community and society as a whole. When we help others achieve their goals and dreams, we strengthen our self-confidence through a sense of accomplishment and purpose.

Inspiration can come from different sources, such as books, lectures, movies, real-life stories of people, or even personal experiences. The diversity of sources of inspiration reminds us that motivation is within our reach, regardless of the context.

Inspiration is also related to empathy. When we put ourselves in someone else's shoes and understand their struggles and triumphs, we are more capable of inspiring and being inspired by stories of overcoming.

Drawing inspiration and inspiring others can occur in all areas of life, from career and education to relationships and health. Through these inspirations, we strengthen our self-confidence in all important areas.

Inspiration is not something static; it can be a constant source of motivation in our journey. Constantly seeking inspiration keeps us engaged and committed to our goals.

Inspiring others requires authenticity. It is important to share our stories and experiences genuinely because it resonates with people and makes our influence more meaningful.

Inspiration can also be an act of gratitude. When we acknowledge the people who have inspired us and express our gratitude, we strengthen bonds and mutual trust.

Drawing inspiration and inspiring others are practices that mutually nourish each other. By inspiring someone, we perpetuate the cycle of motivation and self-confidence.

Inspiration often comes from personal achievements and triumphs. By recognizing and celebrating our own accomplishments, we can inspire others to pursue their own dreams.

In summary, inspiration is a vital component in building and maintaining self-confidence. It motivates us to pursue our goals, strengthens our values, and builds meaningful connections with others. By drawing inspiration and inspiring others, we nurture a virtuous cycle of motivation and self-confidence that helps us overcome challenges and achieve our dreams. This chapter is an invitation to seek inspiration in your life and recognize the power of inspiring others as a powerful way to strengthen your self-confidence.

CONCLUSION

As we reach the end of this book, I hope you have found inspiration and guidance to strengthen your self-confidence and apply it in all areas of your life. The journey of self-confidence is one of the most important we can undertake, as it is the key to achieving our dreams, overcoming obstacles, and creating a meaningful and fulfilling life.

Throughout the pages of this book, we have explored various aspects of self-confidence, from understanding its nature to practical application in real-life situations. We have covered topics such as the importance of self-confidence, discovering your inner self, overcoming insecurities, exploring passions and talents, strategies for boosting self-confidence, facing obstacles, and celebrating personal achievements. Additionally, we have addressed how self-confidence relates to interpersonal relationships, work, and career.

Along this journey, you have discovered that self-confidence is not an innate gift reserved for a lucky few, but rather a skill that can be cultivated and improved over time. It requires self-awareness, self-compassion, and the willingness to face challenges with determination. Self-confidence is not the absence of fear but the courage to act despite fear. It is believing in yourself, even when doubt tries to creep in.

The importance of self-confidence cannot be overstated. It influences every aspect of our lives; from the decisions we make to how we relate to others. It is a critical factor for success, personal fulfillment, and happiness.

Remember that self-confidence is an ongoing journey. It can grow and strengthen as you nourish it with positive actions, self-acceptance, and learning from experiences. At times, you may face setbacks, moments of self-criticism, and challenges that test your self-confidence, but these are opportunities to grow and become even stronger.

Throughout this book, you have also learned about the importance of self-care, mutual inspiration, and maintaining self-confidence throughout life. These are essential aspects to sustain your self-confidence and continue reaping the benefits it offers.

Remember that the journey of self-confidence is personal and unique to each individual. Your experiences, challenges, and achievements shape your journey uniquely. Do not compare yourself to others but seek your own growth and development.

Our journey to self-confidence is a quest for the best within us. It is a commitment to believe in our talents, pursue our dreams with determination, and build healthy and rewarding relationships. It is the journey to become the most confident and authentic version of ourselves.

As you close this book, I want to remind you that self-confidence is a quality that resides within you. It is yours to nurture and cultivate. Continue to believe in yourself, pursue your goals with determination, and inspire those around you with your journey of personal growth.

May this book have provided the tools and inspiration needed for you to move forward on your journey with renewed self-confidence. Always remember that you are capable of achieving everything you desire when you believe in yourself. Move forward with courage and confidence, for the world is ready to witness the power of your self-confidence.

ABOUT THE AUTHOR

Ike Baz is the pseudonym of a Brazilian writer. Graduated in Mathematics in Brazil and with a postgraduate degree in Education in Portugal, Ike Baz is a world explorer, having visited more than 20 countries, including intriguing destinations like India, Nepal, and Thailand, as well as countries in South America, Russia, various regions of Europe, and the United States of America.

Ike Baz is a tireless inquirer who conducts research in various fields of knowledge, ranging from mathematics, physics, psychology, philosophy, history, technology, astronomy, and human behavior. A true enthusiast of lifelong learning, he believes that knowledge is a powerful tool for understanding the world around us. Through his travels and studies, he seeks to enrich his worldview and share valuable insights with his readers. His goal is to inspire others to also explore the vast universe of knowledge and embrace intellectual adventure. With an open mind and a passion for discovery, Ike continues his journey of exploration and learning, eager to unravel the mysteries that the world has to offer.

www.ingramcontent.com/pod-product-compliance
Lightning Source LLC
Chambersburg PA
CBHW050743260726
48661CB00001B/380